SPOTLIGHT ON GLOBAL ISSUES

MENTAL HEALTH FOR ALL

Jill Keppeler

ROSEN PUBLISHING
NEW YORK

Published in 2022 by The Rosen Publishing Group, Inc.
29 East 21st Street, New York, NY 10010

First Edition

Editor: Theresa Emminizer
Book Design: Michael Flynn

Photo Credits: Cover FatCamera/E+/Getty Images; (series globe background) photastic/Shutterstock.com; p. 4 Chanintorn.v/Shutterstock.com; p. 5 Lapina/Shutterstock.com; p. 7 Mita Stock Images/Shutterstock.com; pp. 8, 9 Print Collector/Hulton Archive/Getty Images; p. 10 Stock Montage/Archive Photos/Getty Images; p. 11 Encyclopedia Britannica/Universal Images Group/Getty Images; p. 12 Library of Congress/Corbis Historical/Getty Images; p. 13 Alfred Eisenstaedt/The LIFE Picture Collection/Getty Images; p. 14 kate_sept2004/E+/Getty Images; p. 15 Monkey Business Images/Shutterstock.com; p. 17 Rich Polk/Getty Images; p. 18 Florent Vergnes/AFP/Getty Images; p. 19 Sumy Sadurni/AFP/Getty Images; p. 21 Manuela Durson/Shutterstock.com; p. 22 kittirat roekburi/Shutterstock.com; p. 23 LightField Studios/Shutterstock.com; p. 25 Marla Aufmuth/Getty Images; p. 26 Neilson Barnard/Getty Images; p. 27 Shannon Finney/Getty Images; p. 29 Wavebreakmedia/iStock/Getty Images.

Library of Congress Cataloging-in-Publication Data

Names: Keppeler, Jill, author.
Title: Mental health for all / Jill Keppeler.
Description: New York : Rosen Publishing, [2022] | Series: Spotlight on global issues | Includes index.
Identifiers: LCCN 2020003529 | ISBN 9781725323445 (paperback) | ISBN 9781725323476 (library binding) | ISBN 9781725323452 (6 pack)
Subjects: LCSH: Mental health--United States--Juvenile literature. | Mental illness--United States--Juvenile literature. | Mentally ill--Treatment--United States--Juvenile literature.
Classification: LCC RA790.6 .K47 2022 | DDC 616.8900973--dc23
LC record available at https://lccn.loc.gov/2020003529

Manufactured in the United States of America

CPSIA Compliance Information: Batch #CSR22. For further information contact Rosen Publishing, New York, New York at 1-800-237-9932.

CONTENTS

CHAPTER ONE

A STATE OF WELL-BEING

When you think of problems that affect the world today, it can feel overwhelming. With environmental issues such as climate change and pollution and social problems such as inequality, education issues, and poverty, it seems there's a lot to worry about. In fact, that can lead back to yet another concern: that of mental health.

Mental health is more than just a lack of mental disorders or disabilities. The World Health Organization (WHO) calls it "a state of well-being in which an individual realizes his or her own abilities, can cope with the normal stresses of life, can work productively, and is able to make a contribution to his or her community." Mental health is an important part of overall health.

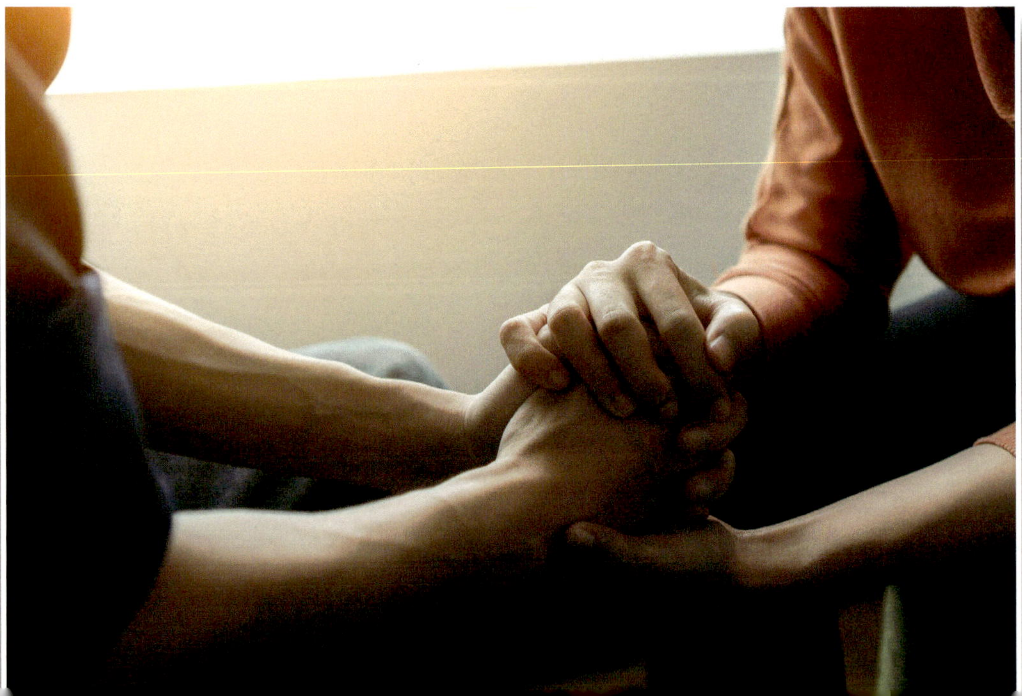

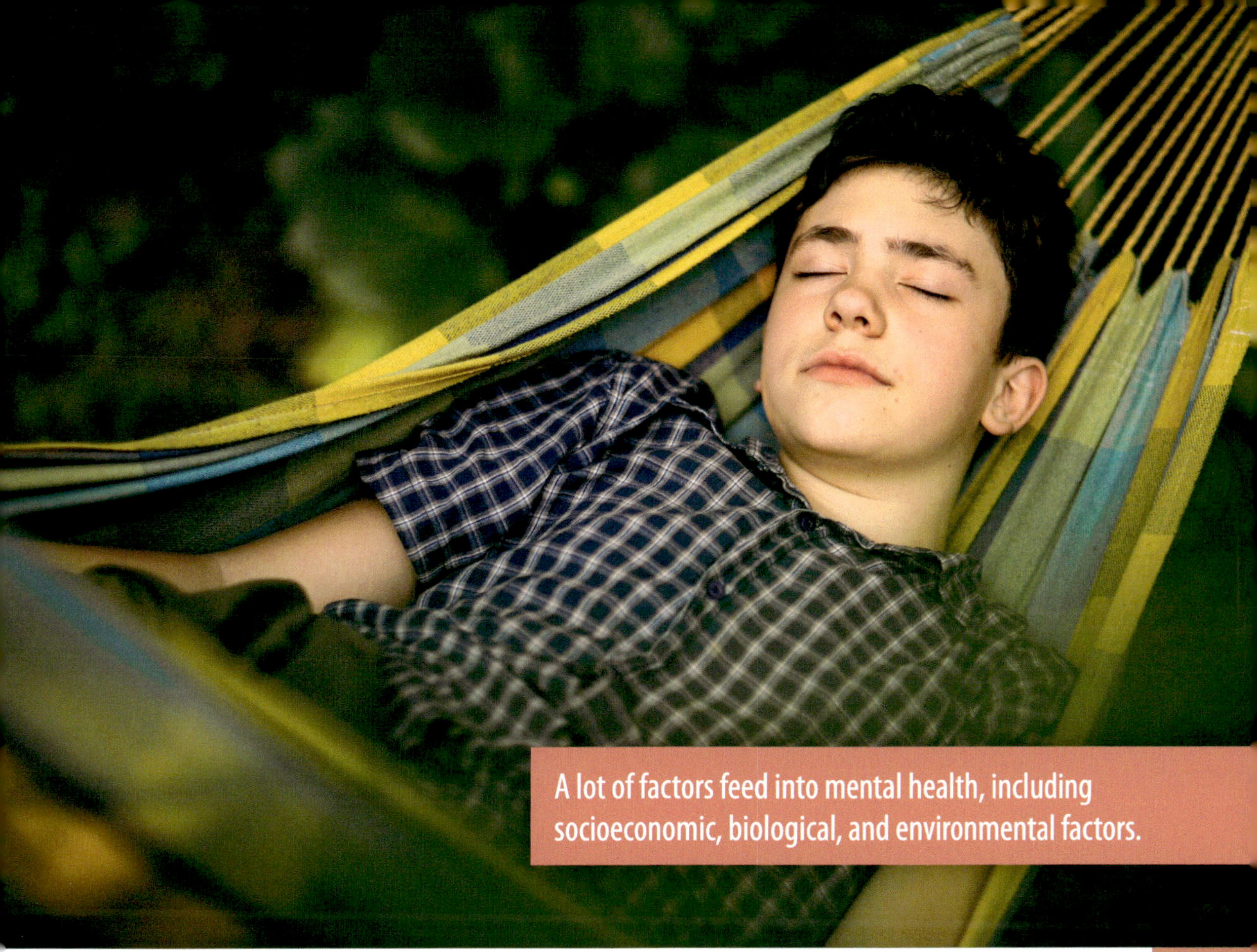

A lot of factors feed into mental health, including socioeconomic, biological, and environmental factors.

Many people today agree that there's a mental health crisis in the United States and the world. This crisis could take a heavy toll on people's lives, as well as on productivity and the world economy. In fact, in 2018, a group of specialists said it could cost $16 trillion between 2010 and 2030 if not addressed.

However, many people are working to help their fellow citizens of the world, drawing attention to problems and coming up with solutions. Activists of all ages are working against the stigma that can come with mental health issues and spreading information about getting help. In fact, you can do your own part to help out too! It's important to be educated and aware about mental health.

While mental health involves more than just mental disorders, these issues are a crisis as well. WHO estimates that one in four people will deal with a mental or neurological disorder in their lifetime. About two-thirds of these people won't receive care for their disorder, whether that's because of the stigma of mental health issues, lack of access to care, or discrimination. Many never even seek care.

In the United States, about one in five adults will deal with mental illness. In fact, one in 25 will experience serious mental illness, according to the National Alliance on Mental Illness (NAMI). About 17 percent of young people ages 6 to 17 also deal with mental health problems.

Mental illness can include many things. Anxiety disorders are the most common mental disorders throughout the world and in the United States, while depression is the leading cause of disability worldwide. They're often connected. Other disorders include bipolar disorder, post-traumatic stress disorder (PTSD), obsessive-compulsive disorder (OCD), and schizophrenia.

Many people might not think of addiction or alcohol and substance use disorders as mental health issues, but they are. They're brain diseases that affect a person's actions. People may often have one of these diseases and other mental illnesses.

Autism spectrum disorders are neurological and developmental disorders. They're not mental illnesses, but they are related to mental health.

Another health issue connected to mental health is suicide. About 90 percent of the almost 1 million people who die by suicide each year have a mental health issue.

If you or a friend or family member are dealing with mental health issues, you're not alone. Help is out there.

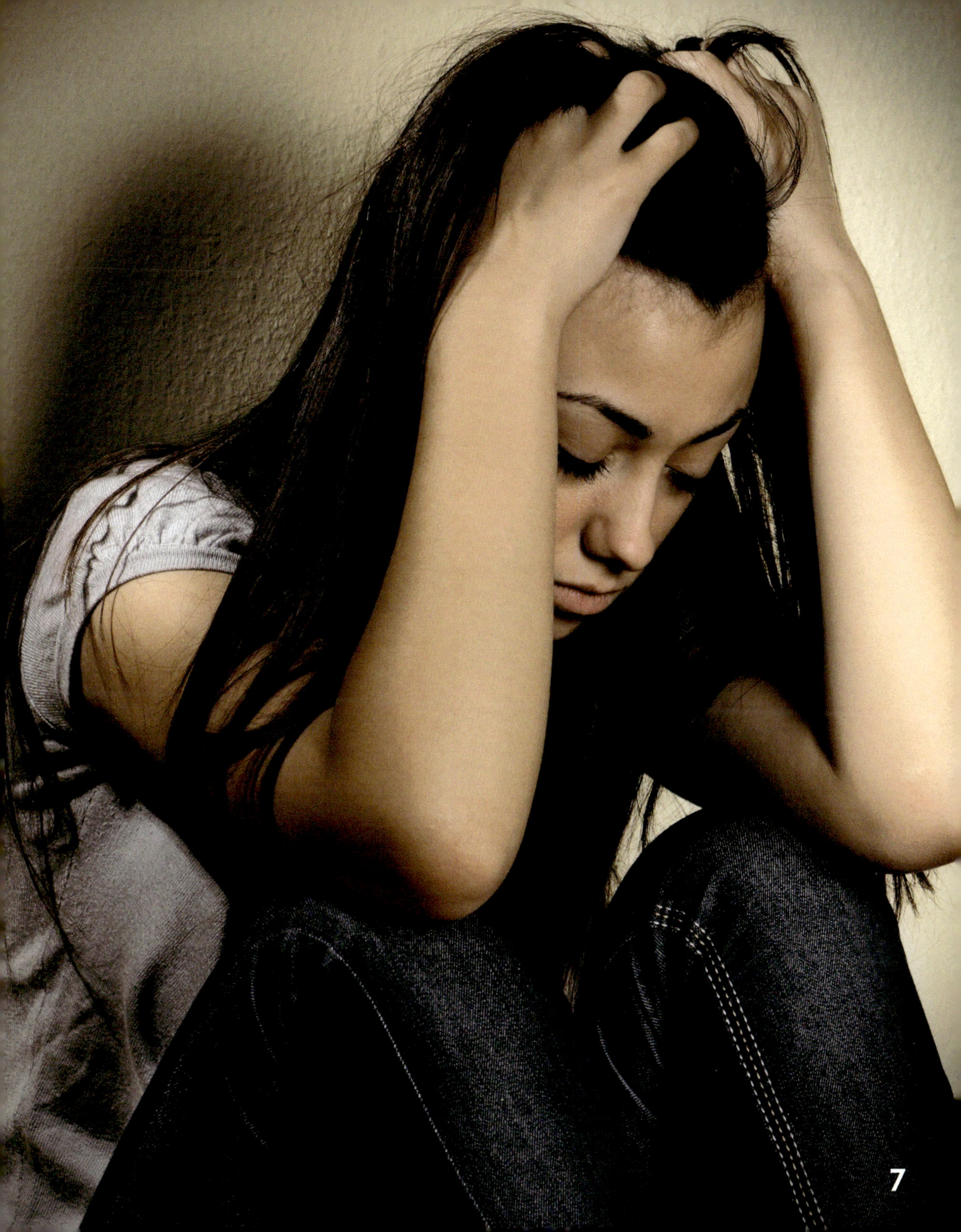

CHAPTER TWO

MENTAL HEALTH AND HISTORY

Although the world does have a mental health crisis, some things have improved over the years. Those with mental health problems were once treated with neglect and outright cruelty. Even those who tried to care for the mentally ill often used inhumane methods. Many people once believed that mental issues had supernatural origins, such as demonic possession. A focus on witchcraft in the 15th to 17th centuries in Europe and the North American colonies increased this belief.

People would sometimes use exorcism, or the practice of expelling a supposed evil spirit by religious figures, to try to help. Trephining, or drilling into a patient's head to release evil spirits, was another method. People treated this way often died.

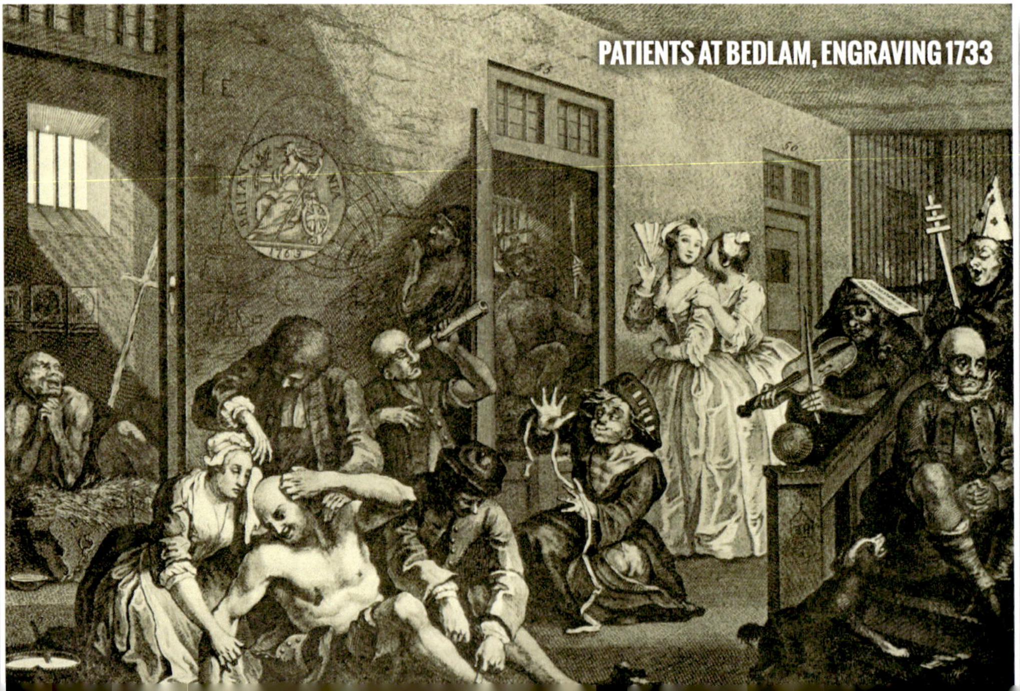

PATIENTS AT BEDLAM, ENGRAVING 1733

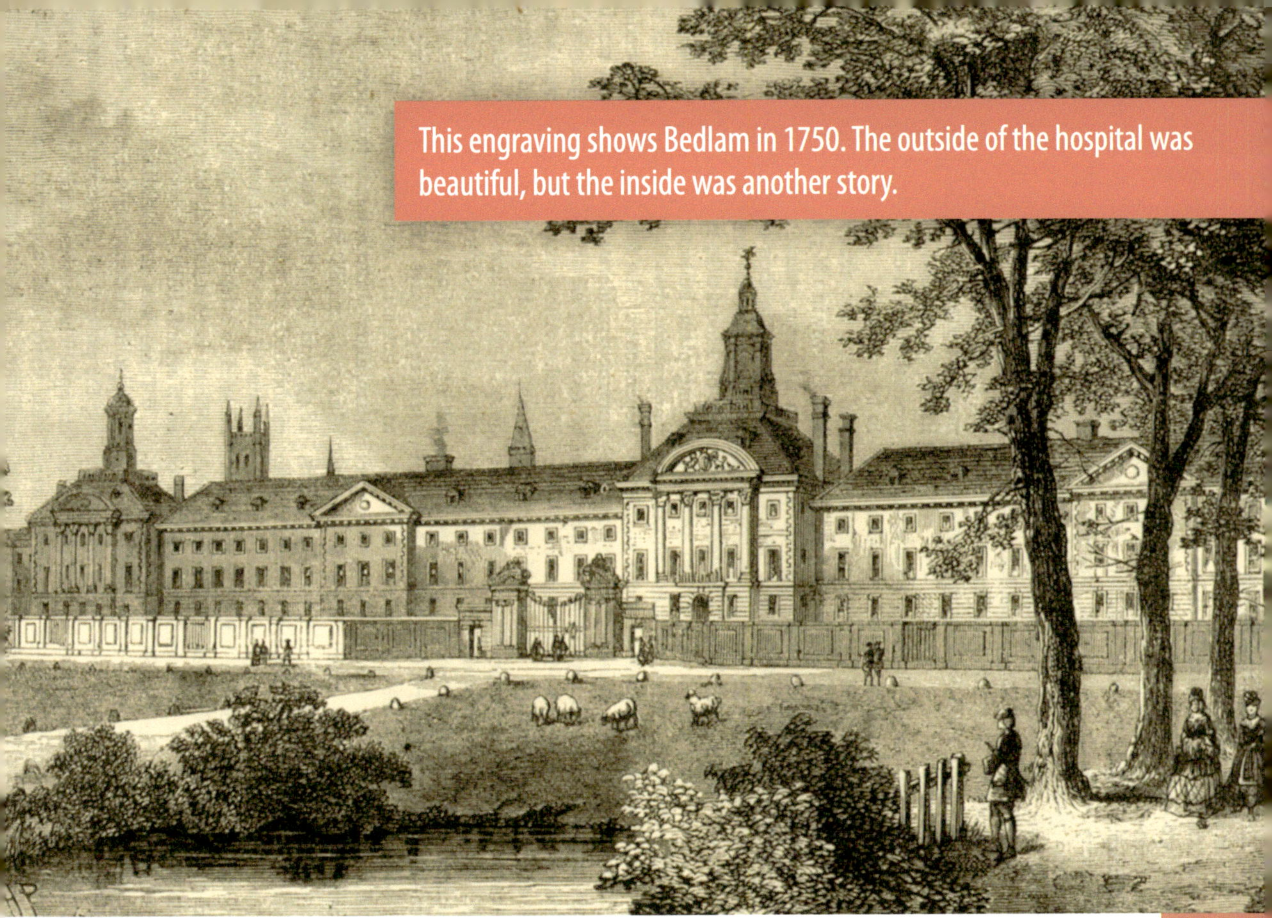

This engraving shows Bedlam in 1750. The outside of the hospital was beautiful, but the inside was another story.

However, not all earlier societies used these means. The Arab region created the first-known mental hospitals in AD 918 in Baghdad and in Cairo. Some Hindu and African cultures also have treated those with mental health issues with more understanding.

However, later European "madhouses," as they were called, were more prisons than hospitals. Bedlam (otherwise known as Bethlem Royal Hospital), founded in London in 1247, was infamous for the harsh way its "patients" were treated. There, and at other such places, patients were often tied up and treated as if they had no feelings at all. The focus was on keeping them away from so-called normal people. However, in the 1600s and 1700s, people could actually pay to go to Bedlam and watch the patients as if they were animals in a zoo.

During colonial times in the area that would become the United States, people with mental issues didn't fare much better. Courts ordered them to be driven from towns or sent them to almshouses, or poorhouses. Sometimes, communities would even auction, or sell, them off, allegedly to be cared for by others. However, they were often exploited in these situations. The first asylum, or institution to care for the mentally ill, in the future United States opened in 1773 in Virginia.

Slowly, some attitudes began to change. In the late 1700s, Philippe Pinel, a French doctor, made the first attempts at real therapy for people with mental health problems. He removed the chains from some of his patients at the Bicêtre, an asylum in Paris, France, shocking others. Some of those patients had been chained up for 30 to 40 years.

Around the same time, William Tuke, an English businessman, started to push for better treatment of people in such institutions. He founded the York Retreat in 1796. It treated patients in humane ways and tried to help them. In the United States, Benjamin Rush, a doctor and a signer of the U.S. Declaration of Independence, also fought for more humane treatment.

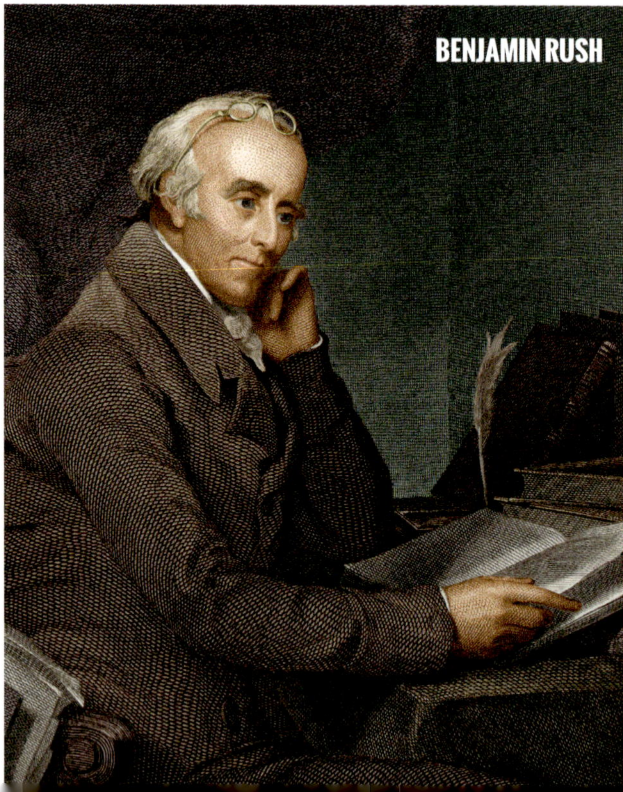

BENJAMIN RUSH

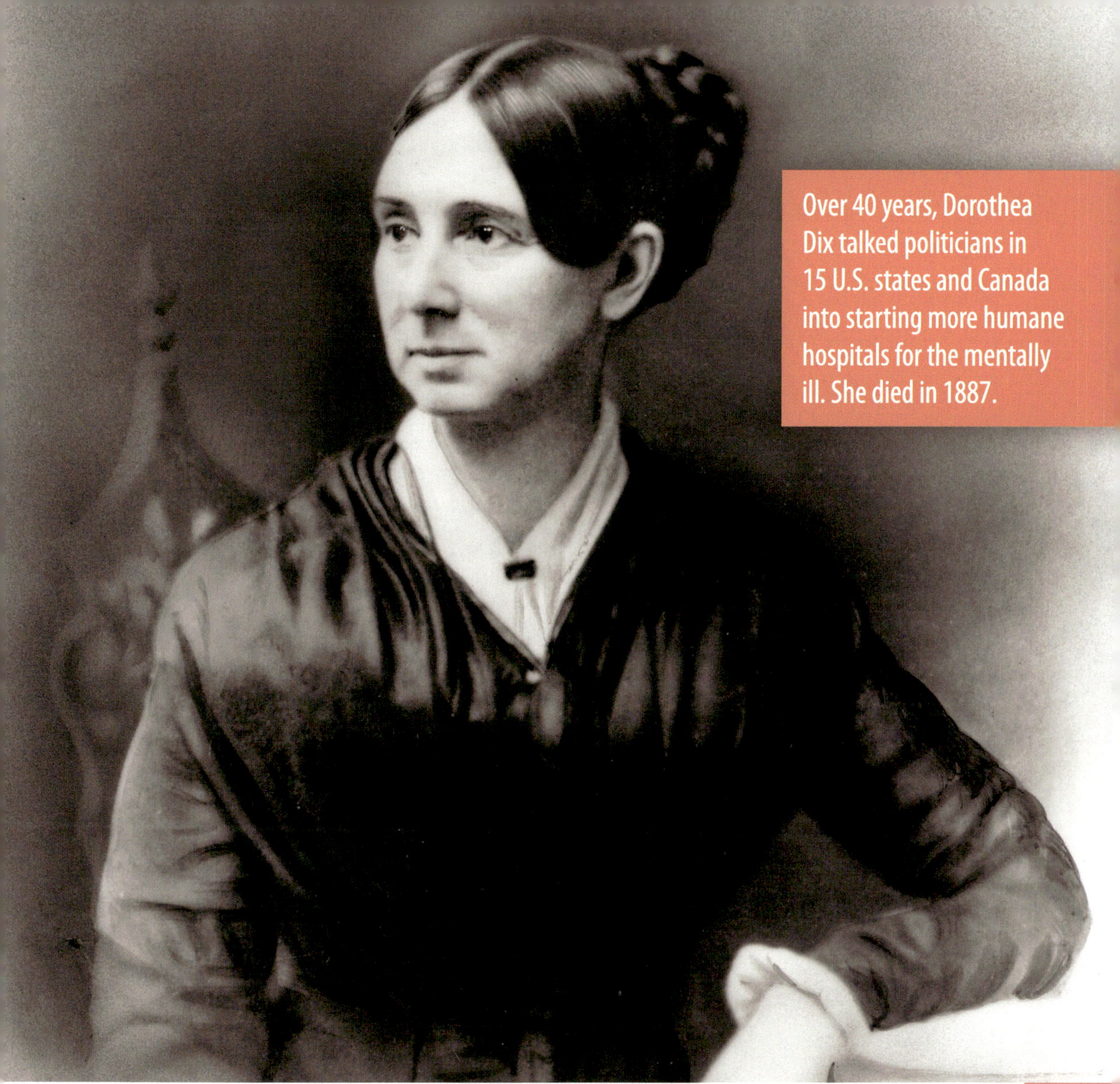

Over 40 years, Dorothea Dix talked politicians in 15 U.S. states and Canada into starting more humane hospitals for the mentally ill. She died in 1887.

One of the most famous campaigners for the rights of the mentally ill was Dorothea Dix, born in 1802 in Maine. A teacher, Dix was horrified to find out that that people with mental disorders were locked up in prisons with criminals and treated in cruel and brutal ways. She began working for reform.

As the world moved into the 1900s, views on mental health continued to change. In 1908, Clifford Whittingham Beers published *A Mind That Found Itself*, his autobiography. It told of his experiences with anxiety and depression—and also of how he was treated badly and abused at a number of mental institutions. He called for more reform for mental health practices and more research into related sciences, such as psychology. This was the start of the modern mental health movement.

However, there were still many ups and downs to come. The mental health movement got a boost after World War II, when many veterans returned home with issues such as PTSD. In 1946, the U.S. Congress passed the National Mental Health Act. This led to the creation of the National Institute of Mental Health (NIMH) in 1949. This organization still exists today.

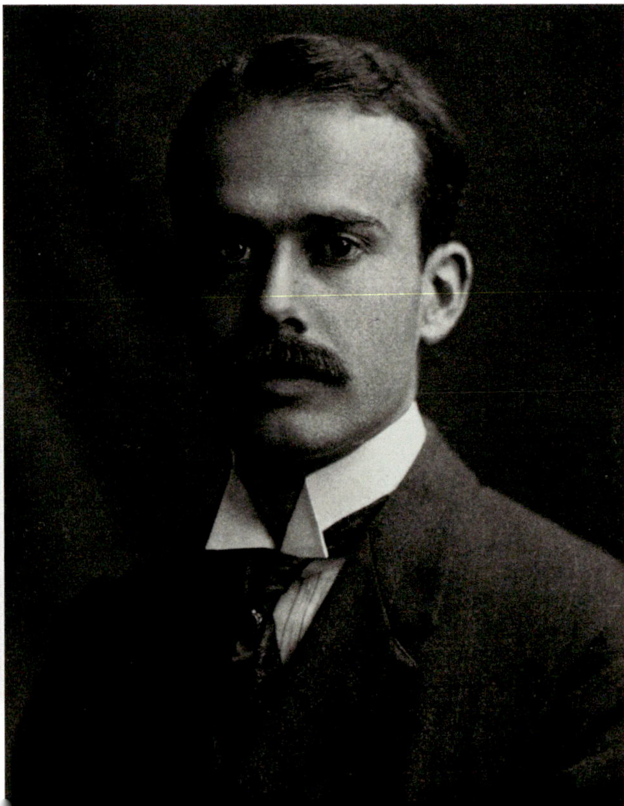

Clifford Beers also helped form the Connecticut Society for Mental Hygiene, the first group of its kind. He later helped create the American Foundation for Mental Hygiene in 1928 and other groups.

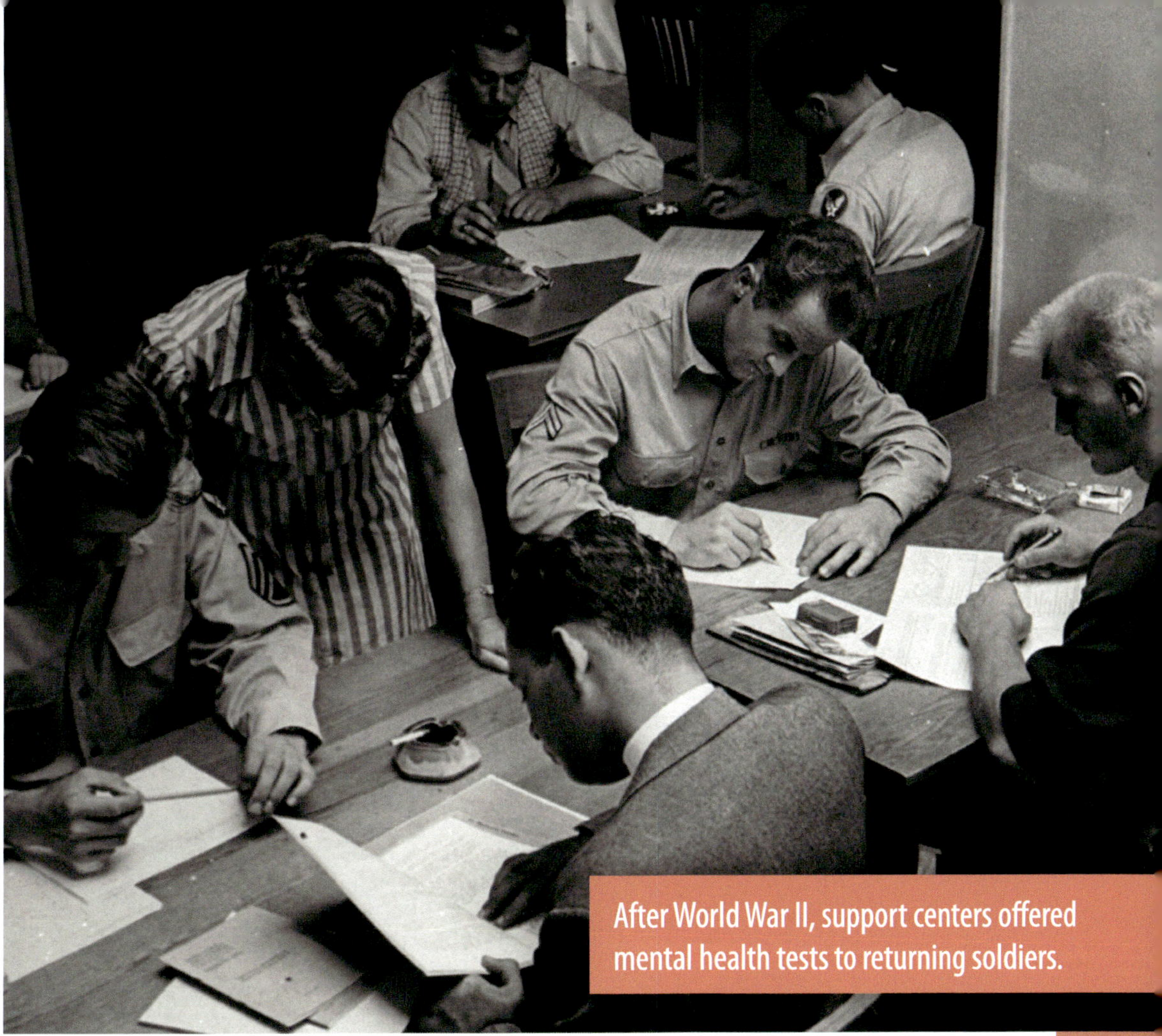

After World War II, support centers offered mental health tests to returning soldiers.

By the 1950s, many mental health advocates pushed for treatment to move away from institutions and more toward community and individual care. By the 1960s in the United States, many institutions closed. In some ways, this helped people, but it also led to lack of care for some people who needed it. Many people with mental issues became homeless. Many also wound up in the prison system. This problem continues today.

Today, much of the focus is on dealing with the stigma surrounding mental health and illness and making sure people have access to the care they need, which may include therapy and medications.

CHAPTER THREE

CROSSING ALL LINES

Mental health issues cross all lines of human experience. They can affect young people, old people, people of all genders and sexual orientations, and people of all different races, ethnic groups, and locations. However, some groups are more affected than others for various reasons.

In the United States, the population is becoming more and more diverse. By 2044, more than half of all Americans are likely to belong to a minority group. Many groups have similar rates of mental health issues, but the effects for some are longer lasting. For example, Black and Hispanic Americans have lower rates of depression than white Americans, but the depression is likely to persist more in those groups for a number of reasons. People who identify as being two or more races are the most likely group to report any mental illness in the past year. American Indians and Alaska Natives are more likely to deal with PTSD or alcohol dependence. However, white Americans die by suicide more than any other ethnic group.

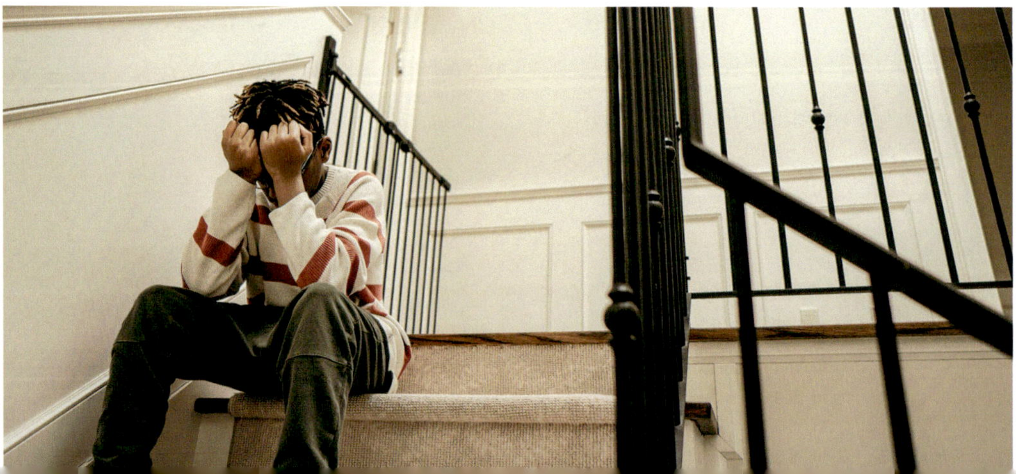

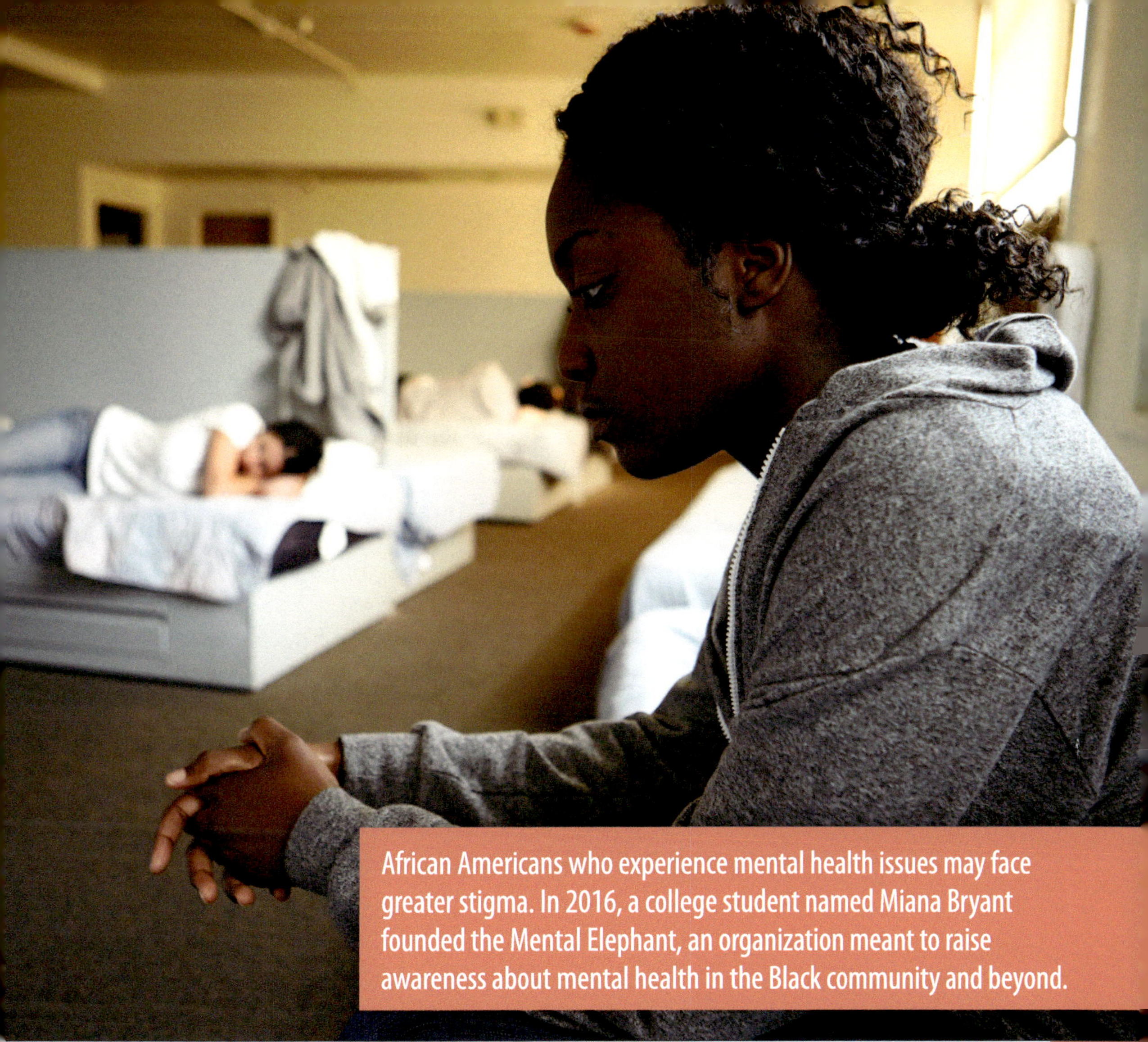

African Americans who experience mental health issues may face greater stigma. In 2016, a college student named Miana Bryant founded the Mental Elephant, an organization meant to raise awareness about mental health in the Black community and beyond.

It can be very difficult to get a clear picture of these issues, though. For example, health-care providers may diagnose fewer cases of mental illness in people from more diverse populations for reasons that include language barriers, cultural differences, and increased stigma of mental illness in different groups. People from minority groups are also less likely to seek care for mental health issues at all. This may be for a number of reasons, including the stigma and poor insurance coverage.

Members of the LGBTQ community may also be affected by mental health issues more than the population as a whole. They may have to deal with a double stigma, both for their gender or sexual identity as well as for any mental disorders. They may have to deal with discrimination, prejudice, and rejection from family or other support groups.

Lesbian, gay, or bisexual adults are twice as likely to deal with a mental health condition as heterosexual adults. LGBTQ people are at much higher risk for suicide attempts than others. In fact, nearly 50 percent of transgender adults reported that they'd attempted suicide in the past 12 months, compared with 4 percent of the general U.S. population, according to NAMI.

LGBTQ young people are at special risk. They may deal with bullying and rejection by family. Without family support, they may not be able to access help and health treatment. They may worry that looking for help will out them to their friends and family, even if they're not ready.

More often, however, activists are starting to look at how all these issues collide in the subject of mental health. Ose Arheghan (who uses the pronoun "they") is a young activist from Ohio who was focusing on LGBTQ issues in high school when they noticed how often those issues and mental health issues came together. They joined the youth ambassador council of the Trevor Project, a national nonprofit that helps LGBTQ young people. Arheghan continues to work for change while a student at Ohio State University.

In 2017, activist Ose Arheghan received the Student Advocate of the Year award at the GLSEN Respect Awards in California.

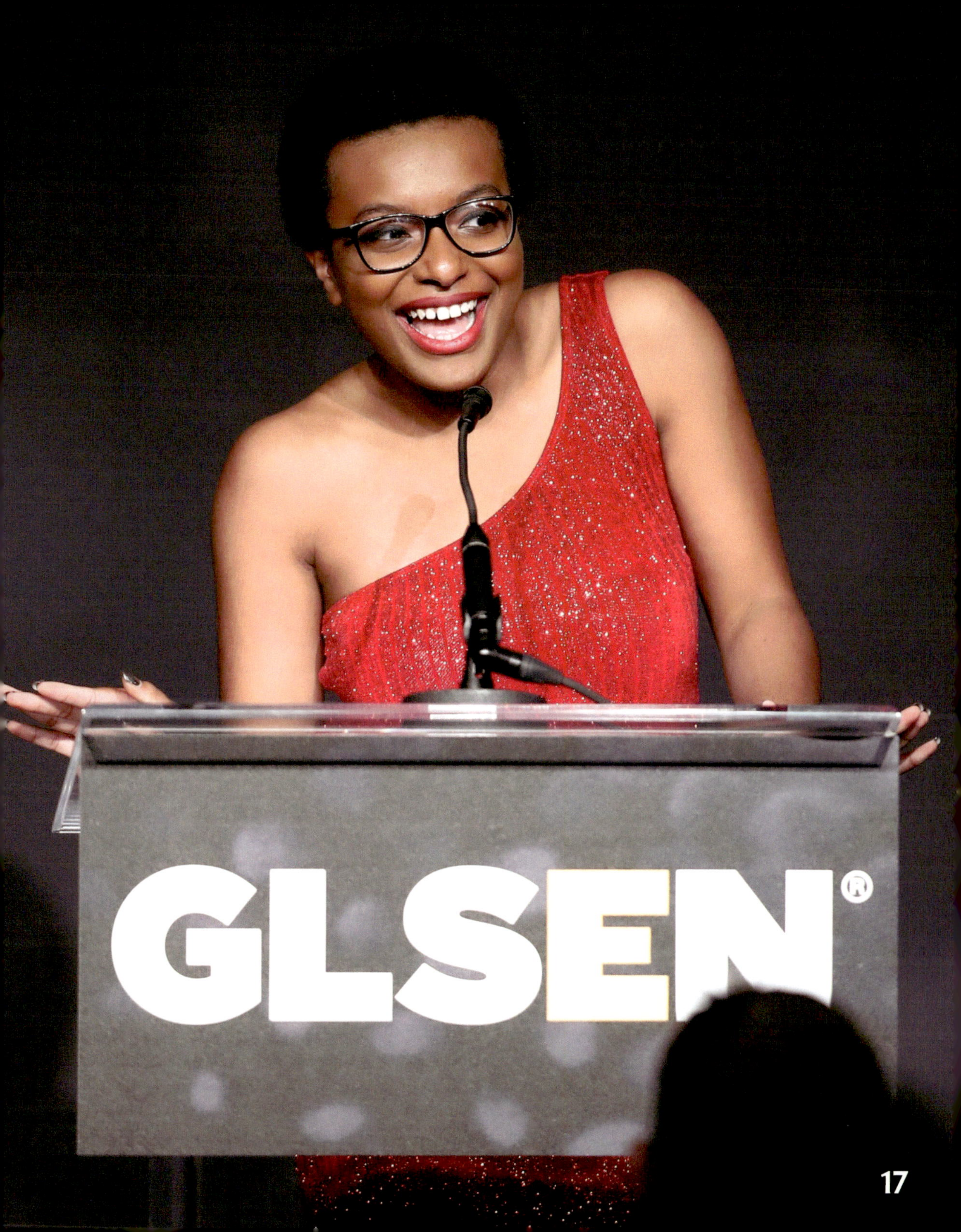
GLSEN

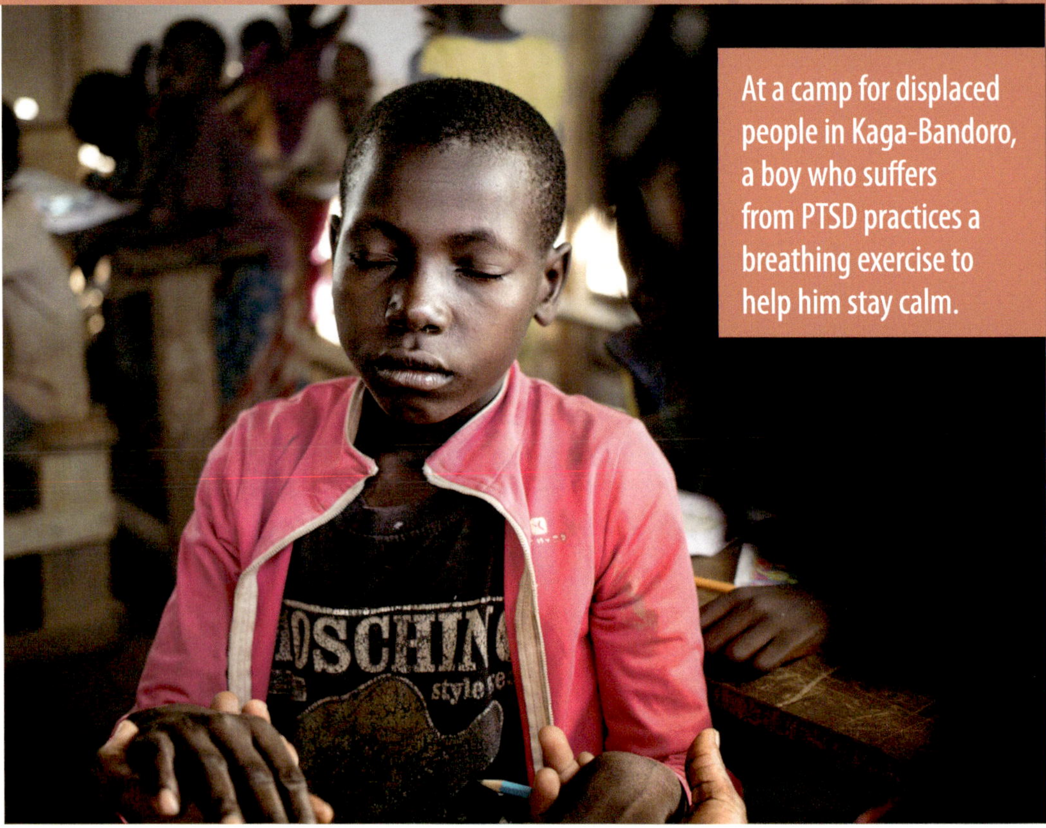

At a camp for displaced people in Kaga-Bandoro, a boy who suffers from PTSD practices a breathing exercise to help him stay calm.

Worldwide, mental health care can be even more complicated. According to WHO, more than 40 percent of countries have no mental health policy, and about 25 percent of countries have no mental health laws at all. More than a third of countries dedicate less than 1 percent of their health budgets to mental health, and about another third spend only 1 percent on mental health. In many countries, there's also a lack of access to medicines used to treat mental health disorders.

There's also a lack of mental health professionals in many places. They make up only 1 percent of the global health-care workforce. According to the American Psychiatric Association, nearly half of the world's people live in a country with less than one psychiatrist per 100,000 people.

In addition, people in countries wracked by war or natural disasters also have much greater problems with mental health issues. They also have even less access to mental health resources. And in any country, the poor are at greater risk of mental health disorders because of constant exposure to stress, unsafe living conditions, poor general health, and lack of access to care.

Activists are working to help. In 2018, Pavel Reppo created mindfullwe (now Finemind), a nonprofit program to help the problem of mental health care in low-income communities. Workers created a community mental health program in Uganda that had many successes. Reppo was inspired to start his work by his own experiences dealing with OCD.

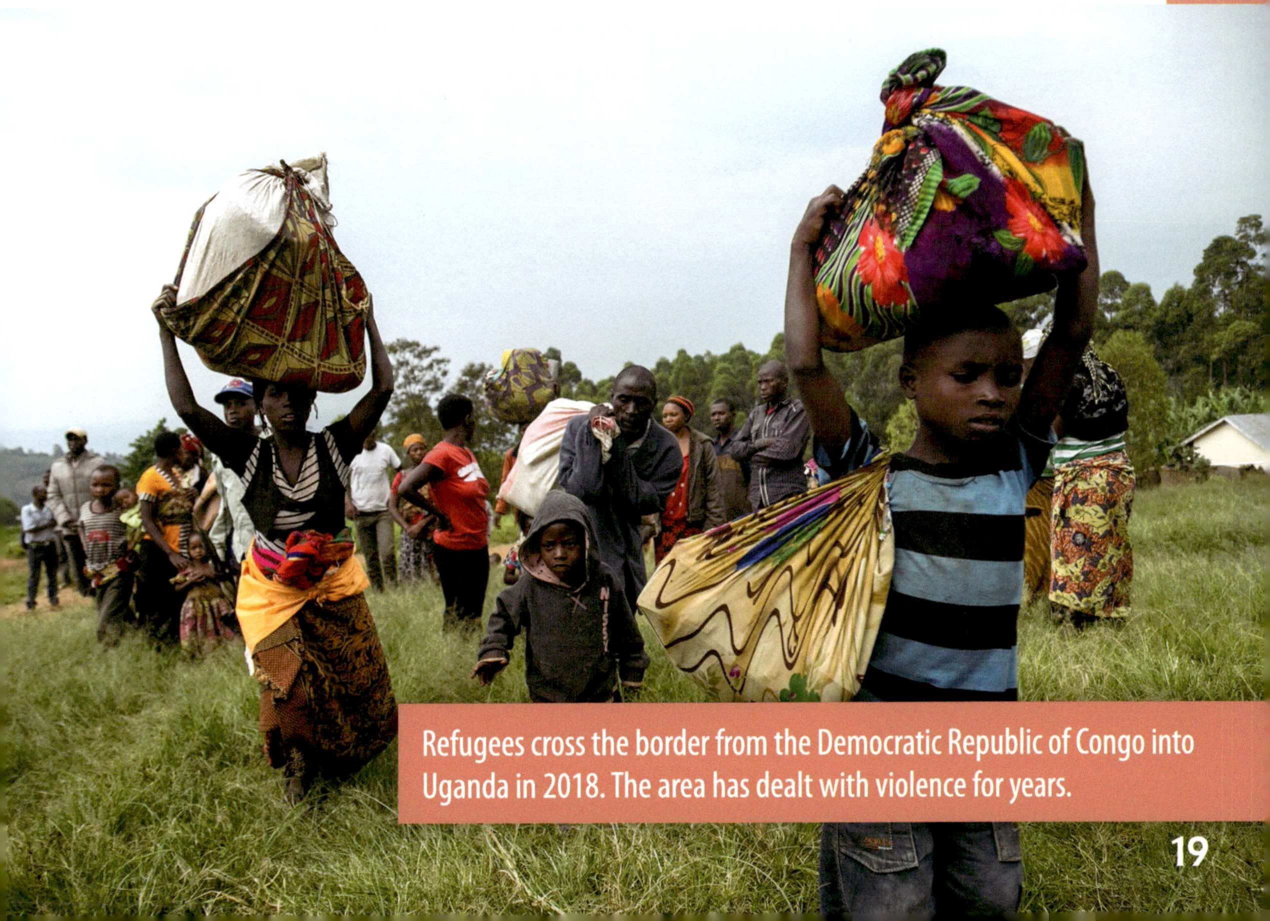

Refugees cross the border from the Democratic Republic of Congo into Uganda in 2018. The area has dealt with violence for years.

CHAPTER FOUR

THE RIPPLE EFFECT

Mental health issues and disorders have a greater effect on people and society than just those issues alone. They have a ripple effect that affects people in many ways and spreads to others.

According to NAMI, people with a serious mental disorder can be more likely to get other serious, chronic illnesses. They also have an increased rate of heart disease. Nearly 20 percent of adults with a mental illness also have a substance abuse issue.

Those who are caregivers to people with mental illness also have their own issues to deal with. They can deal with a lot of stress, and many may become depressed. More than 8 million Americans alone provide care to someone dealing with a mental or emotional illness, according to NAMI. It can take a mental toll, and it can also be a lot of work, taking time away from the person's job and other family members. It can have a serious effect on entire families.

Suicide resulting from mental illness also has a huge ripple effect. In the United States, it's the 10th leading cause of death—and the second leading cause of death for people ages 10 to 34. The overall U.S. suicide rate has increased by 31 percent since 2001.

A person's suicide not only affects family members and friends but also community, church, and school members. It can even affect those who never personally knew the person who died, such as emergency response personnel and those who help the family afterward.

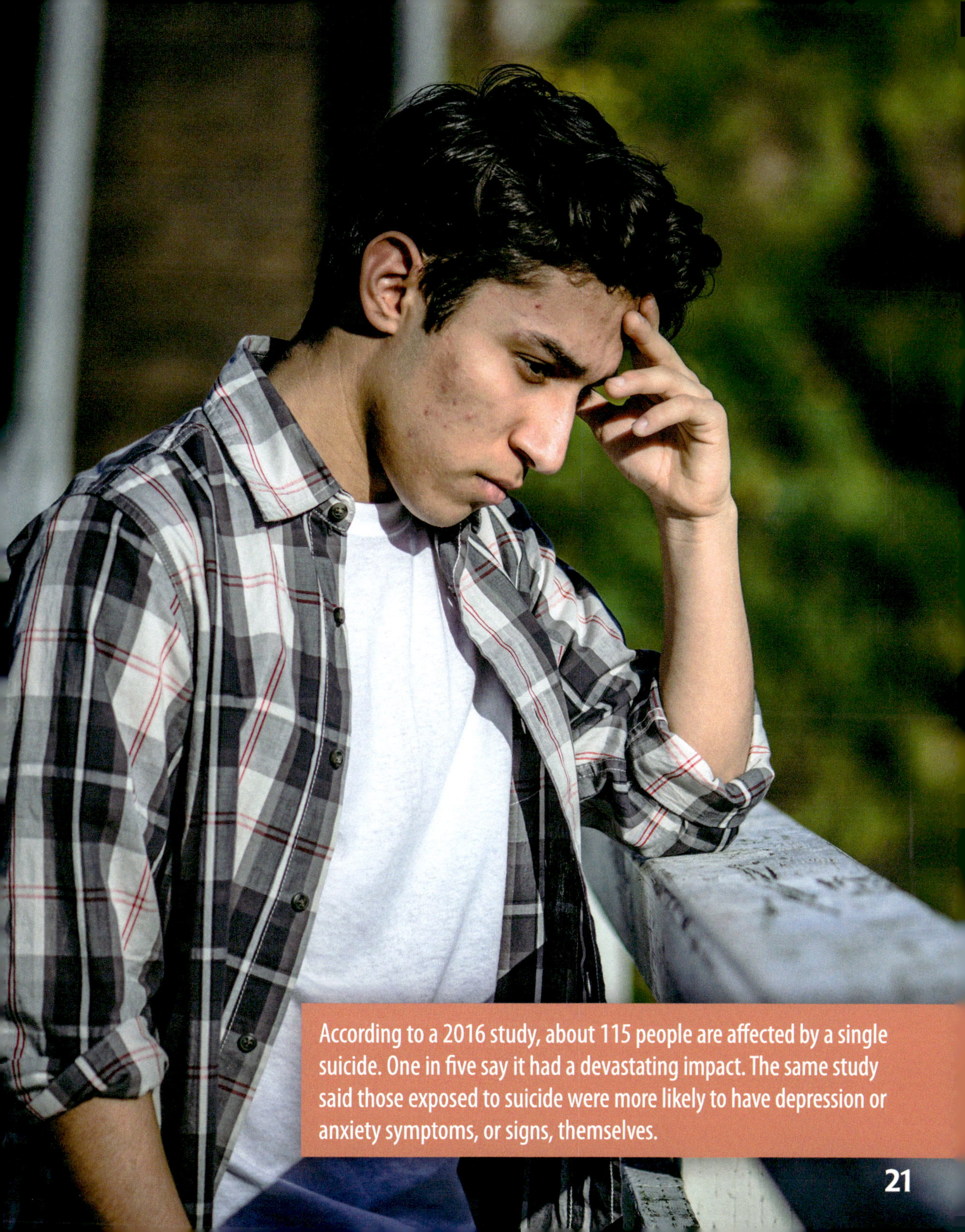

According to a 2016 study, about 115 people are affected by a single suicide. One in five say it had a devastating impact. The same study said those exposed to suicide were more likely to have depression or anxiety symptoms, or signs, themselves.

Mental health makes ripples in other ways too. According to NAMI, about a fifth of people who are homeless in the United States have a serious mental health issue. Nearly 40 percent of those in the state or federal prison system have a diagnosed mental health disorder, and 70 percent of those in the juvenile justice system have a mental health problem as well.

Most inmates with mental health issues are nonviolent offenders. However, while people are in prison or other systems, they're not likely to get the care they need, so they may get worse instead of better. And after they leave jail or prison, they're likely to have lost the means to get mental health care. Some may end up homeless or repeat the cycle.

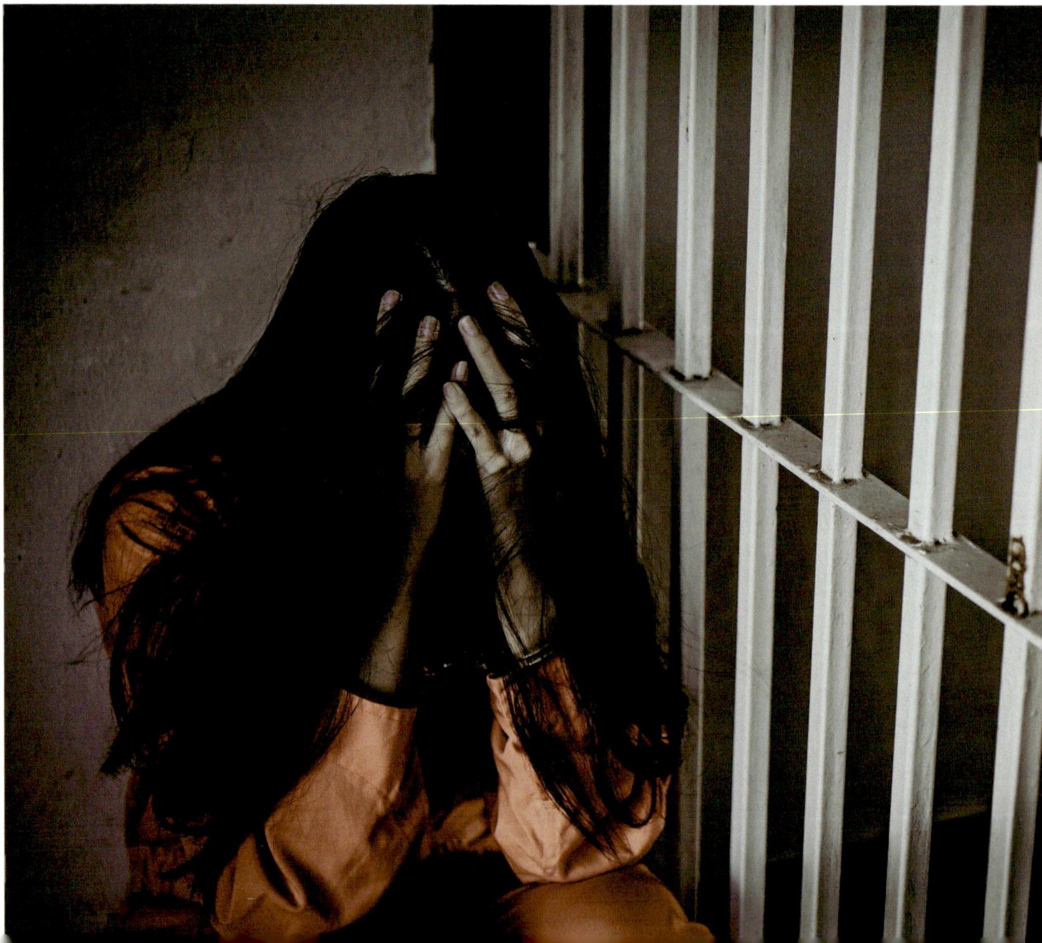

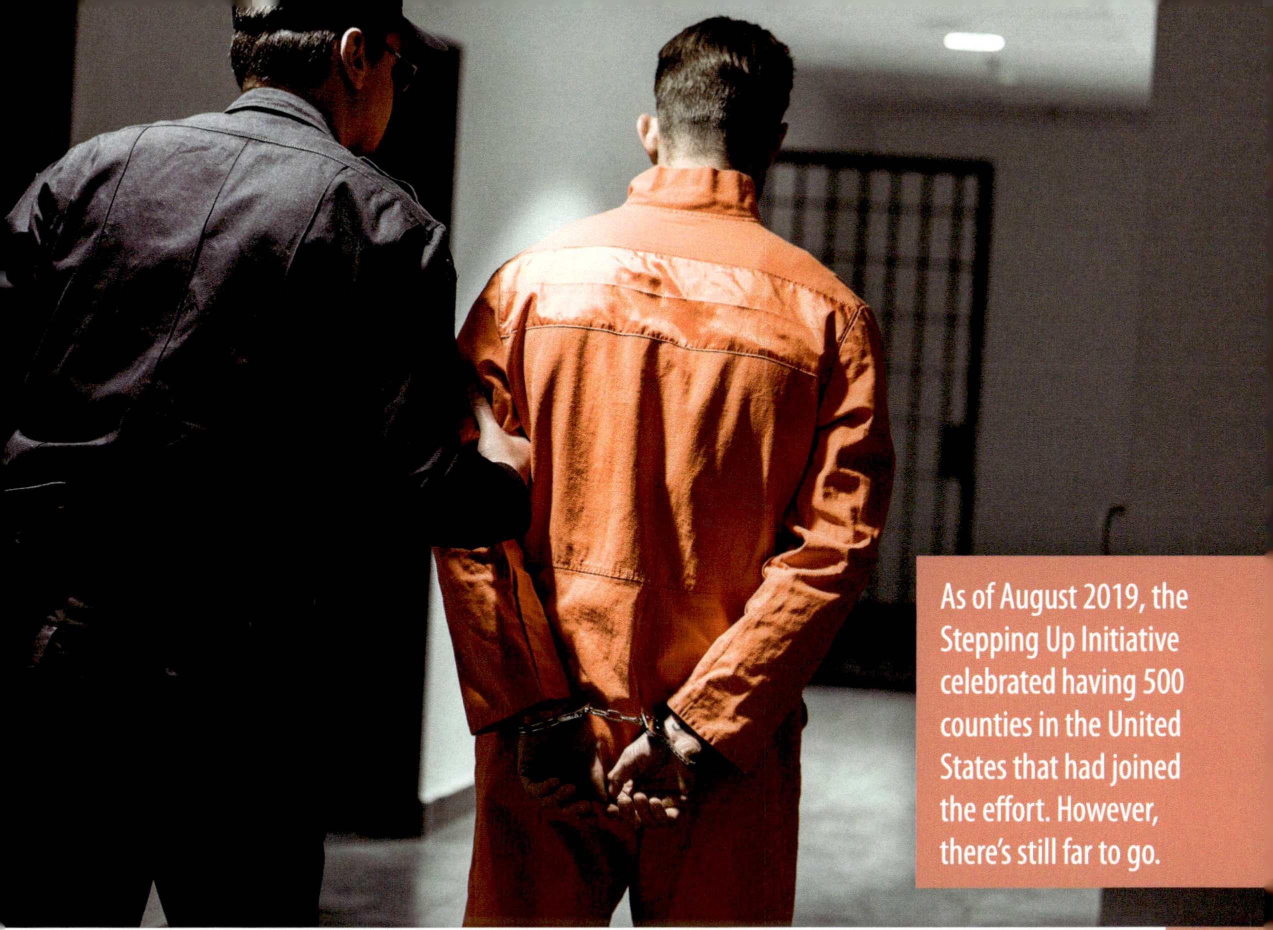

As of August 2019, the Stepping Up Initiative celebrated having 500 counties in the United States that had joined the effort. However, there's still far to go.

This also has an economic effect. According to the Stepping Up Initiative, a national effort to keep people with mental illness out of jails and get them into treatment, jails spend two to three times more money on adults with those illnesses. However, this often doesn't help either the inmates or public safety in any real way. And it puts more pressure on institutions that already tend to be underfunded.

The Stepping Up Initiative is helping train criminal justice professionals to identify people with mental illness and respond in a better way, directing those people to groups that can help. It's also working to connect people already in jail with mental health services. The organization includes state and local leaders, criminal justice and health professionals, and people who have mental illnesses.

CHAPTER FIVE

MAKING A DIFFERENCE

Including those who take part in the Stepping Up Initiative, many people—including many young people—are coming together to work for mental health awareness. They're speaking out about their struggles and those of others and working to reduce the stigma of mental disorders. They're turning to new technologies to help out, as well.

Amanda Southworth of Los Angeles struggled with her mental health in middle school and high school. She was only 13 years old when she created the app AnxietyHelper, which gives young people tools and resources to help them deal with anxiety and mental health. The app has since been downloaded more than 3,000 times, and it has more than 1,000 regular users.

Since that, Southworth has created more apps (including Verena, a security app for the LGBTQ community) and started her own nonprofit software development company, Astra Labs. She was also named one of *Teen Vogue*'s 21 Under 21 for 2017.

"Everything in my life has shown me that both good and bad things in this world will continue to happen and that's out of our control," Southworth said in a TedX talk in November 2017. "But it's what we do with the things that happen to us that can make all of the difference."

Southworth isn't alone in her use of coding to make a difference. Satvik Sethi, a student at Binghamton University in New York State, created Runaway, an app on which people can talk with volunteers. He also helps organize mental health awareness events.

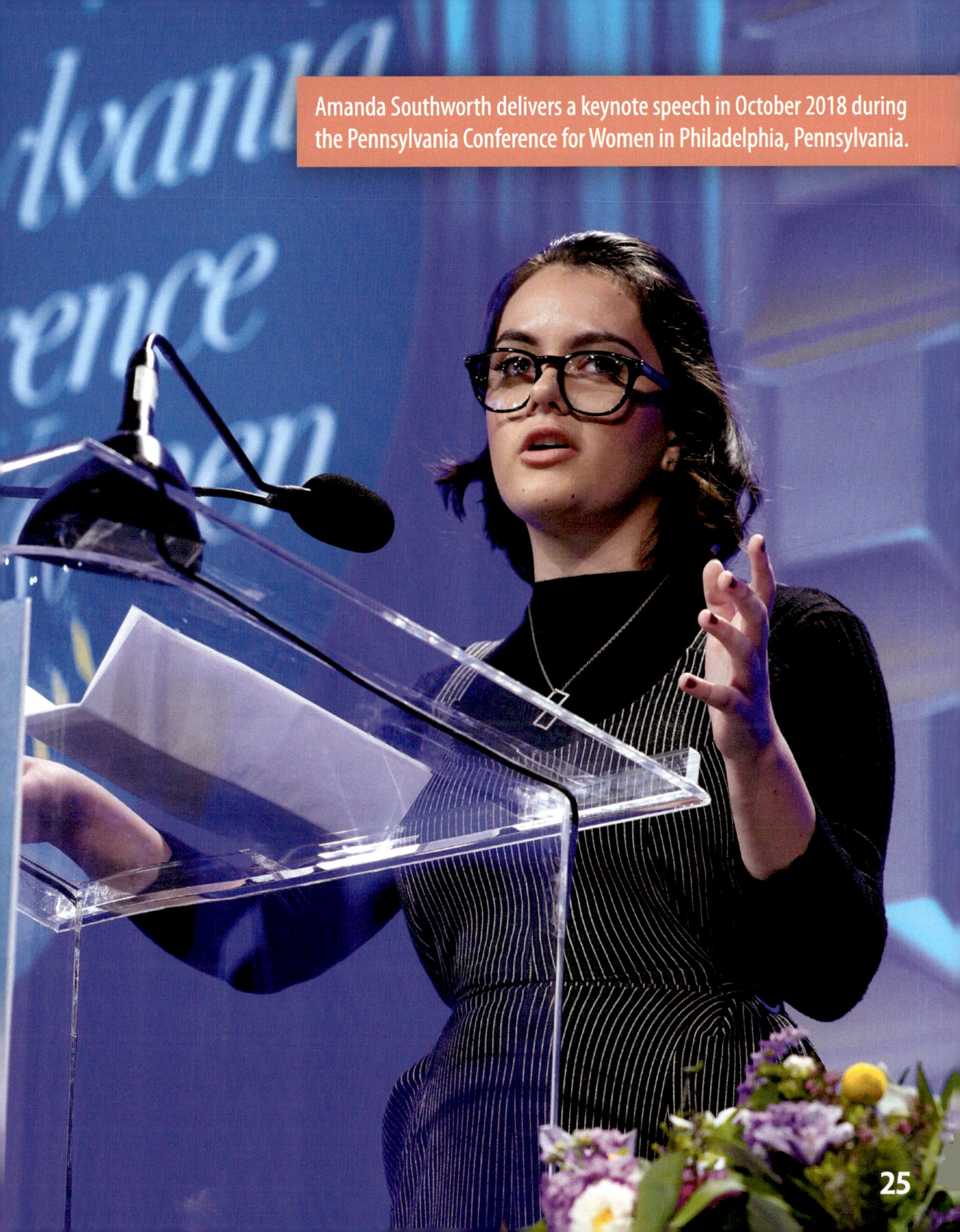

Amanda Southworth delivers a keynote speech in October 2018 during the Pennsylvania Conference for Women in Philadelphia, Pennsylvania.

Many young activists work as part of bigger groups—or create their own. Or both!

Lehlogonolo Muthevhuli, a young activist in South Africa, is working for equal rights to health care and more mental health awareness there. She's also a member of the Amnesty International Global Youth Collective, working for human rights worldwide.

Gabby Frost of the United States founded the Buddy Project in 2013, when she was 14. The campaign, now a nonprofit organization, aims to help prevent suicide by pairing people at risk with buddies to support them. More than 200,000 people have signed up to be a buddy since 2013.

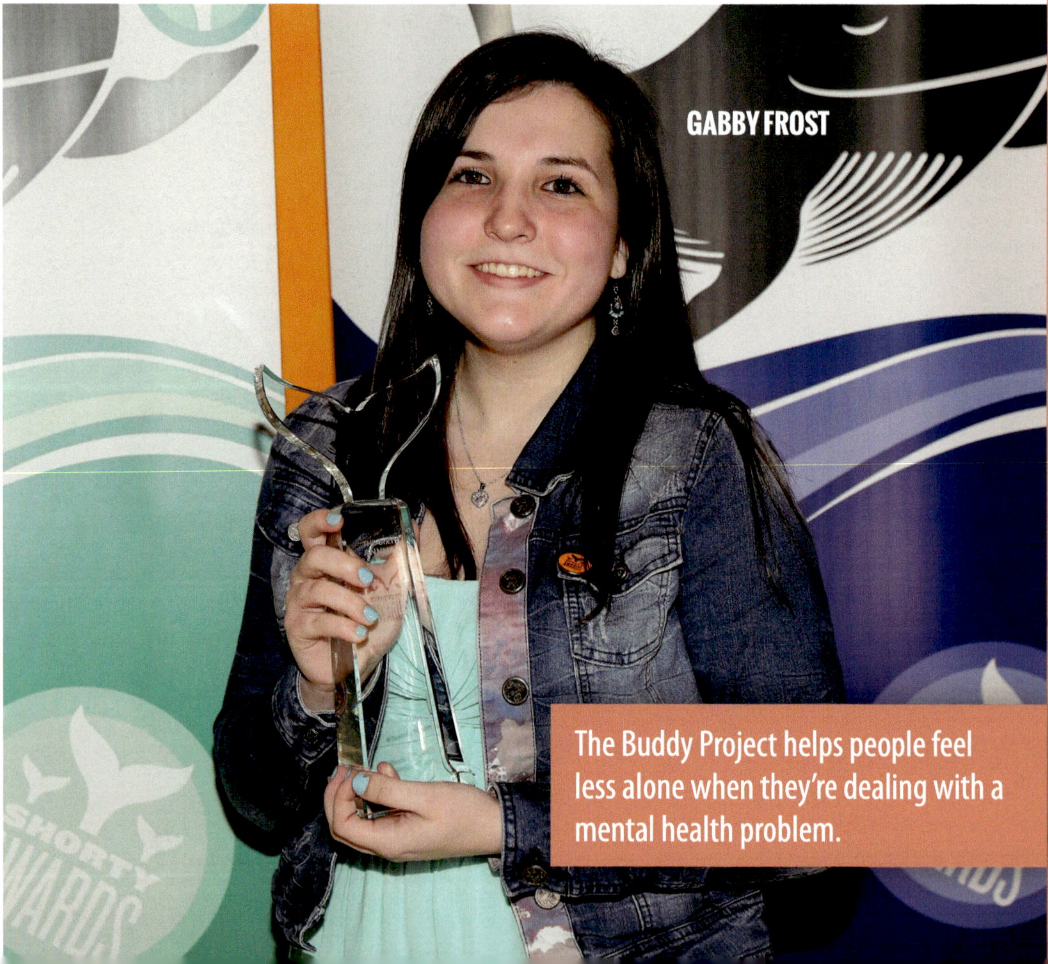

GABBY FROST

The Buddy Project helps people feel less alone when they're dealing with a mental health problem.

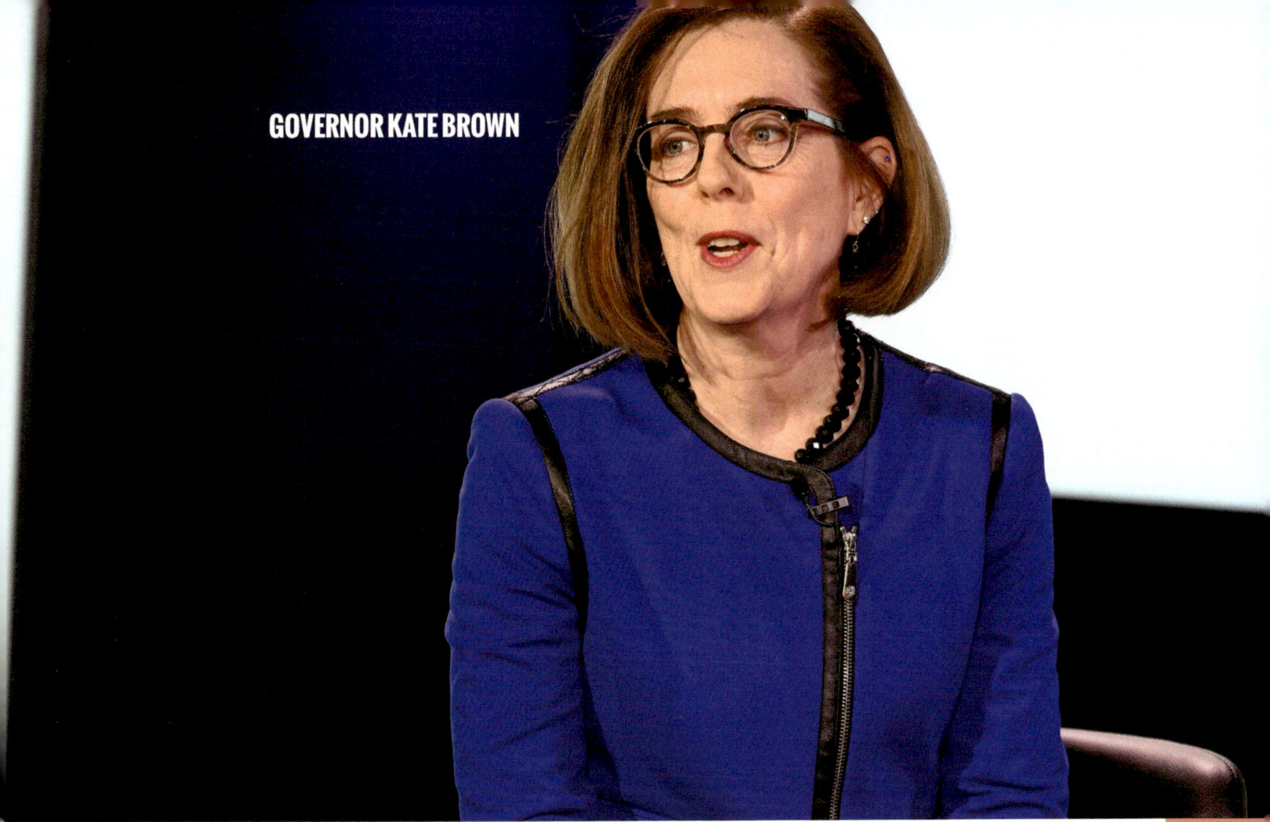

Hailey Hardcastle of Oregon and other teen activists campaigned for a state law to allow students to take excused days off from school when they're dealing with mental health issues. Governor Kate Brown signed it into law in June 2019.

"We're not talking about 'I just don't feel like going to school,'" Chris Bouneff, executive director of NAMI in Oregon, told NPR. "We're talking about real disorders, real things that have real impacts." Bouneff said the law encourages students to be honest and could help with awareness and acceptance.

Many young activists work with school or campus groups. Sam Orley was a student at the University of Michigan when he became the director of the Wolverine Support Network, one of the country's first college peer support groups. The WSN is now expanding its model to high schools and colleges through the United States.

So, what can do you to support mental health awareness and well-being? You can help break the stigma about mental health issues by taking NAMI's stigma*free* pledge (www.nami.org/stigmafree), which has people promise to learn more about mental health, teach others about mental health, avoid judging those with mental illness, and take action to support mental health.

If you've dealt with a mental health issue yourself, you can share your story. Be sure to talk to your parents first to be sure you're not sharing information that's too personal.

You can avoid using words such as "crazy" or "insane" as insults. Use words that are kind and that aren't judgments about mental health issues. Watch out for bullying at school and take steps to stop it, either by stepping in or by telling someone you trust.

You can also watch for friends at school who seem to be dealing with depression or anxiety and offer them support and understanding. Notice signs of trouble such as losing interest in things they used to like or talking about feeling hopeless. Encourage them to talk to you. The Embrace the Awkward campaign online offers suggestions to start a conversation with a friend about mental health. It notes that you don't have to be an expert to start a talk—just be a friend.

If you know someone who threatens suicide, be sure to tell a trusted adult as soon as you can. If the problem is immediate, you can call 911 in the United States.

Starting a conversation about mental health can be awkward—but you can do it!

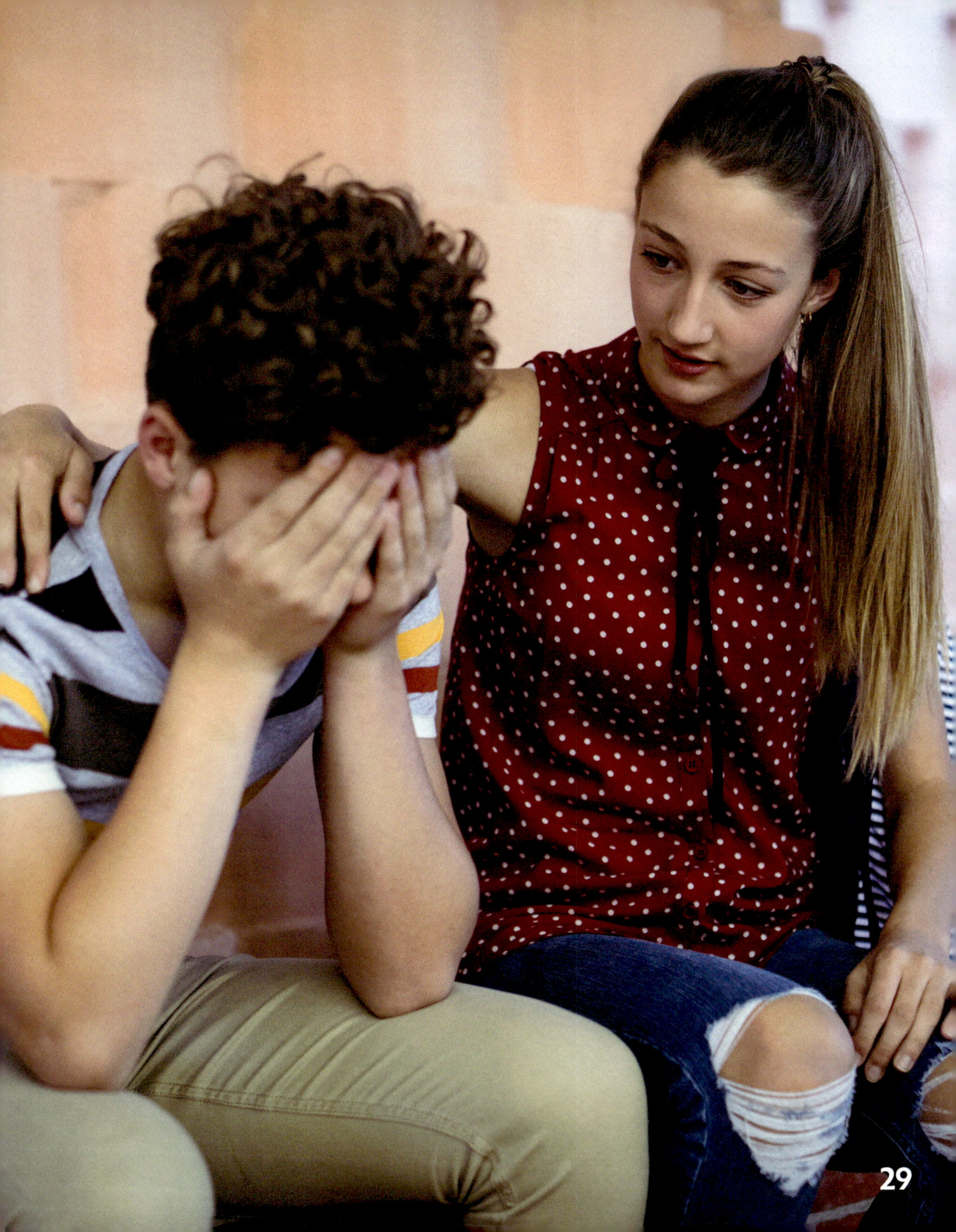

CHAPTER SIX

IN THE FUTURE

There's a mental health crisis in the world today, but there's also much hope. If we work to make sure the stigma about mental health issues fades, there will be even more chances to get people the help they need.

Technology may also help with global mental health. People having mental health issues can speak with a therapist or crisis center simply by texting or using an app. Some therapies can be delivered online to those who don't have access to other means of help. Some future apps may even be able to sense an upcoming mental health crisis from a person's behavior online or in other ways. Some apps may teach coping skills. Others may track symptoms. Apps can also help researchers collect information about mental health.

There's a long way to go in the quest for better mental health care, but there are encouraging signs. In the future, there may be more of a focus on dealing with mental health issues before they happen instead of just dealing with them after the problem has started. That may delay issues or outright prevent them and keep the problem from growing.

Younger generations, often more comfortable with talking about mental health, are leading the charge. Today's young activists are working to build on the work of those who went before them, break stigmas, encourage conversations, and create new technologies to help themselves, their peers, and their world. With advocates like this, the future is full of hope indeed.

GLOSSARY

activist (AK-tih-vist) Someone who acts strongly in support of or against an issue.

advocate (AD-vuh-kuht) A person who argues for or supports a cause or policy.

autism (AW-tiz-uhm) A developmental disorder that can affect social interactions, thoughts, and behaviors.

chronic (KRAH-nik) Continuing or occurring again and again for a long time.

crisis (KRY-suhs) An unstable or difficult situation.

demonic (dih-MAH-nik) Relating to a demon, or an evil spirit.

diagnose (diy-ihg-NOES) To identify a disease by its signs and symptoms.

discrimination (dih-skrih-muh-NAY-shuhn) Different—usually unfair—treatment based on factors such as a person's race, age, religion, or gender.

diverse (diy-VUHRS) Having many different types, forms, or ideas.

ethnic (ETH-nik) Belonging to a certain group of people who have a culture that is different from the main culture of a country.

exploit (ek-SPLOIT) To use someone in a way that helps you unfairly.

inhumane (ihn-hyu-MAYN) Not kind or good to people or animals.

neurological (nuhr-uh-LAA-jih-kuhl) Having to do with neurology, or the scientific study of the nervous system and the diseases that affect it.

psychiatrist (suh-KIY-uh-trist) A person who practices a branch of medicine that deals with mental, behavioral, or emotional disorders.

socioeconomic (soh-see-oh-eh-kuh-NAH-mihk) Relating to a combination of social and economic factors.

stigma (STIG-muh) A set of negative, often unfair beliefs that a society or group of people have about something.

suicide (SOO-uh-siyd) The act of killing oneself.

technology (tek-NAH-luh-jee) A method that uses science to solve problems and the tools used to solve those problems.

therapy (THER-uh-pee) A way of dealing with problems that make people's bodies and minds feel better.

INDEX

PRIMARY SOURCE LIST

Page 9
Bethlem Royal Hospital, also known as Bedlam. Colored engraving. About 1750. Now held by the Wellcome Collection.

Page 11
Dorothea Lynde Dix. Deguerreotype. About 1850 to 1855. Samuel Broadbent. Now held by the Boston Athenaeum.

Page 17
Ose Arheghan at 2017 GLSEN Respect Awards. Photograph. October 20, 2017. Rich Polk. California. Now held by Getty Images.

WEBSITES

Due to the changing nature of Internet links, Rosen Publishing has developed an online list of websites related to the subject of this book. This site is updated regularly. Please use this link to access the list: www.powerkidslinks.com/SOGI/mentalhealth